OW TO BE HEALTHY AND IVE LONGER

ought to you by:
y Walkins B.S., CFT

Walkins holds a B.S. Degree in Exercise Sciences, Nutrition and is a
tified Fitness Trainer

hor of:
w to Start a Running Routine and Become a Confident Runner (A Beginner's Guide to
ining and Jogging)

d

Walkins's Fitness Knowledge

Table of Contents

Section One

The Basic Principles of Longevity

As more and more scary facts are revealed about what we consume every day, and what we are doing to ourselves, more and more people are reconsidering how they live their lives. They start looking at the damage being done, and where it might lead to.

Unfortunately, the sad reality is that if you continue to apply unnecessary pressure to your body or mind *(or both, since one affects the other)*, you are likely to vastly reduce the quality of your life as you start getting older.

Once upon a time, aging was associated with numerous aches and pains, with the body showing the signs of all the beatings it had to endure during its productive years.

However, thanks to the availability of modern day knowledge, there is no need for that any more.

By paying some attention to your body and its needs, and respecting its limitations, you can preserve the quality of your life for many years to come, and grow old gracefully, rather than pathetically.

At the end of the day, increasing your chances at longevity is a choice - *yours*.

Key Areas to Living Longer

While there are a multitude of topics could be included when discussing longevity, there are a few basic key areas of your life that should be singled out as vital components:

1. Are you taking care of what you have? Are you still hammering your body into delivering what you want from it, rather than accepting what is reasonable?

. What are you eating? You are what you eat - and you are what you on't eat. What you consume makes a huge difference to what your life vill be like when you grow older.

. Are you allowing your environment to stress you out? Stress has caused nany people to grow old long before they were supposed to be.

. Are you still adding unwanted toxins to your system? The less you pay ttention to what you are doing to your body, the sooner it will wear own.

. Are you paying attention to the little things? Are you taking care of your yes, your skin, your feet, etc?

. Are you paying attention to your weight? Excess weight can cause a nultitude of problems - none of which you need to live with.

. Are you an active person? There is a difference between being active nd being disorganized to the point of constantly rushing.

. Are you getting enough sleep? Sleep is not just the time your body akes to rest - it is much more than that.

. Are you taking anything to slow down the natural aging process, like ntioxidants? You have the power to cheat nature, and turn on the rakes.

hese are the questions we'll be answering throughout this book, and opefully by the end of it... you'll be on your way to a healthier, longer asting life.

Are You Taking Care of Your Body?

Many people carry on day by day, simply demanding that their bodies perform at the levels they want them to. In the process, they add such unnecessary amounts of pressure to their systems that they literally wear themselves out too soon.

Water

One key factor which is commonly neglected is the consumption of enough water. While we are regularly reminded by well educated doctor that we need to consume at least eight glasses of water per day, we fail to do so, and only tend drink water when we "feel" thirsty.

Sadly, though, thirst is not a reliable indicator of whether your body needs more water or not. In fact, usually when you feel thirsty your body has already become dehydrated!

Keep in mind that three quarters of your body is actually water. As such, everything in your system revolves around water. This includes digestion and the transport of nutrients, the uptake of oxygen in the lungs, the cleansing of internal organs, the detoxification system, sweating to reduce your internal temperature, the transport of instructions through the nervou system, and even basic activity on a cellular level.

Thirst is just an indication of a lack of water in your mouth, throat, and stomach. The rest does not cause any physical thirst, but it can cause considerable problems if not attended to anyway, including deterioration of the skin, dysfunctional organs, and more.

Joints

Another thing to consider- are you taking care of your joints, or are you simply allowing them to take all the hammering you seem to enjoy throwing at them?

ne of the biggest single causes of aches and pains in older people are
erworked joints - with many of them having to undergo surgery for hip
placements, shoulder socket repairs, etc.

ile hard work - as the proverbial expression states - has never killed
yone, it has caused many people's lives to deteriorate into a living hell.

wer Back

other common cause for concern is the way you treat your lower back.
ile you are young, you fail to acknowledge that we have to grow older
me day, and that we have to live with the aches and pains we cause
rselves.

a result, we try to be strong, or rather show others that we are strong,
picking up and carrying heavy objects, often in ways that cause
rmanent damage to our lower backs. Since the damage happens
adually, you probably don't notice anything until it is already too late.

only have one physical body, and we have to look after it as best as
can, or pay the price later on. Some things can be repaired physically
egardless of the cost involved - but some cannot.

best and simplest way to increase your longevity is to educate
urself about what your body needs, and to take care of it as well as you
ssibly can!

You Are What You Eat

You know, there is an expression that states "You are what you eat- and you are what you do not eat". It's actually quite true!

Once again, however, the ill effects of not eating properly do not show immediately, but only manifest themselves over time.

First, you have to consider what your body needs. In order to function optimally it needs a wide selection of vitamins and minerals, fiber, water and energy.

Consider Supplements
Thanks to modern day advertising, many people are under the impressic that you can do away with natural vitamins and minerals, and simply tak dietary supplements.

Unfortunately, it has been proven that while these supplements are - in most cases - beneficial, there is also plenty of evidence pointing to the fact that they lack some capabilities offered only by their natural counterparts.

Consume Fresh Fruits and Veggies

To ensure your body gets what it needs, you will need to consume fresh fruit and vegetables as often as possible. While the selection itself is most a matter of personal preference, you should really try to include as man different varieties as possible.

Each fruit and vegetable has its own unique selection of nutrients to offe and consuming a variety of these will ensure that your intake of natural nutrients will be well balanced.

Be Careful with Supplements

Another thing to keep in mind is be careful about indiscriminately consuming large amounts of vitamin supplements. While it is true that some vitamins can be taken in rather large quantities without any direct ill effects, there can be consequences.

In some cases, the excess consumption of one vitamin can lead to the suppression of the functions of another. For instance - if you consume too much vitamin A, your body has problems creating vitamin D.

It is a problem that easily arises if you drink many different supplements and the content from the different sources start adding up.

Buy Organic

Finally - go organic wherever possible. It is an unfortunate truth that modern day farming practices were developed around productivity - and that undesirable substances were introduced along the way.

As a result, many common food items that we perceive as fresh and healthy are simply not that healthy any more. Wherever possible, check the source of your fresh food items, and see if they were organically raised.

Avoid Processed Foods and Artificial Sweeteners

Staying away from processed foods goes *(I hope!)* without saying. It has been the root cause of many ailments, ranging from allergies to migraines.

The same goes for any synthetically created sweetener - instead opt for something natural like products made from Stevia *(a natural herb which is 300 times sweeter than sugar in its pure form)* if you need to replace sugar in your diet.

Aspartame - the basic ingredient for most artificial sweeteners - has more than 90 documented negative side effects.

In short, keep it natural and keep it balanced. Here's to living longer!

Are You Allowing Stress to Destroy Your Life?

Being healthy and how you can help yourself live longer, stress has been the cause of a lot medical problems for a lot of people. While many people think that the effects of stress are - literally - "all in the mind", it goes beyond that, and the effects can be devastating.

What most people do not know is that stress was never intended to be a long term condition. Stress was originally intended as a measure to react in "fight or flight" conditions - in other words, life threatening or dangerous situations.

As such, when stress comes to exist, your body starts diverting all possible resources to a few basic organs - which might be needed to flee or fight for survival.

The response was never intended to last for a long period of time, since usually the "fight or flight" situation would be resolved - either way - within a matter of minutes.

Once resolved, everything in your body was supposed to return to normal again within a few minutes *(provided you were still alive!)* but during that time you needed to be able to perform at abnormal levels.

One of these temporary priority changes is the redistribution of water in your body. Water is temporarily diverted from a number of organs to offer ample supply to muscles and lungs.

Additionally, to ensure an ample supply for as long as is needed, water is also withdrawn from the lower back region - which explains why many people suffering from chronic stress will also complain about chronic back pain.

There are a number of things to keep in mind when dealing with stress:

. In many cases, stress is a matter of choice. While it is true that our attitudes determine how we react to stressful situations, it is also true often we create unnecessary stress, or allow others to stress us out. How much stress you experience will partly be a matter of character, and partly a matter of choice. Some things are worth stressing about, and some are not - analyze your unique situation, and decide for yourself.

. Stress is - in many cases - created from being disorganized. If you are not able to discern between what is urgent and what is important, and treat both the same way, you will be creating stress for yourself. Urgent things need to be taken care of as soon as possible, but in as short a period of time as possible. Important tings need to be scheduled, and the proper amount of time devoted to them.

. Many people simply have to live with huge amounts of stress - some of it might be due to their careers, and some of it might be due to circumstance or the environment. If your stress originates from a source you cannot change, find a way to deal with it. Explore different stress-reducing activities, and see what works for you. For some people it is better to indulge in physical activity, and for others it is better to engage in relaxing tasks or hobbies.

Stress is a very real threat to your longevity - so make a point of keeping it down to the absolute minimum. In the end, only you can make the changes necessary for your health and well-being.

Section Five

Are You Still Poisoning Your Body?

Many people are constantly adding undesirable substances to their bodies - some deliberately, and some unknowingly - yet all of them through ignorance. Are you one of these people?

The first category of people introduces harmful substances to their bodies deliberately. These include acts like smoking, drinking excessively, consuming unnecessary pharmaceutical products, substance abuse, indulging in junk food, etc. If you are doing this, you are definitely creating a negative impact on your longevity - regardless of the reason.

Sadly, some of these actions - like smoking, for instance, cause damage to your system that can never be fully reversed, and which you will have to live with forever. As such, every cigarette reduces your chances of ever having a quality life when you grow older.

The second category of people consumes foods that contain undesirable substances - mostly unbeknown to them. They fail to check the ingredients of any packet, and lack the knowledge to discern organic products from products laden with chemicals and hormone supplements, genetically engineered vegetables, and products poisoned using insecticides.

The fact of the matter is that your system can only handle so much in terms of toxins introduced to it. In most cases, your liver has to do the dirty work, followed by the kidneys and the skin *(some unwanted substances are excreted along with sweat through the skin's pores).*

What you might not realize, however, is that our bodies already have to cope with a lot of pollution and allergens already, and any additional introductions simply add to the load. As a result, your system gets to a point where it simply cannot get rid of everything any more, and starts collecting toxins.

Unfortunately, once these toxins have compounded to a certain level, they will start affecting the functioning of your body in general and thus

duce the overall quality of your life. If this happens on a continuous
sis, a number of your organs can be placed under continuous strain,
eating the possibility of premature organ failure.

e only way to stop poisoning your system is to educate yourself. Once
u know what is harmful, and how it damages your body, you will know
at to avoid - and why. Ignorance has a very high price tag - especially
is paid in ill health.

the end of the day, allowing undesirable toxins to enter your body is
gely a matter of attitude. We have all been made aware of their
stence, and we have all been made aware of the dangers.

that means even if you are still consuming toxins due to ignorance, it
n be rectified with a simple change in attitude - from an attitude of "ah,
ll" to an attitude of "let me find out more". It's your choice, do you
oose life?

Section Six

Are You Paying Attention to the Little Things?

In the rush of trying to keep up with modern day life, we often start neglecting the little things. Unfortunately, these little things add up, and eventually they start affecting your quality of life - at a time when you least want to experience it!

Skin

First of all, while many women pay meticulous attention to their skin, some are "simply too busy" to care. For other people, looking good takes preference over taking care and that leads to neglecting the health of their skin.

Surprisingly, it is not only about the face, but about your skin in general that's important. And unfortunately, most men don't even bother, deeming themselves to "manly" to pay attention to the health of their skin.

Sadly, though, your skin is more complex and important than you might realize.

On the physical side, it is your first line of defense against infectious intrusions. If your skin is easily damaged, or repeatedly damaged due to the type of work that you do without adequate protection, you will constantly be at risk for infection.

Additionally, the skin is considered to be "the third lung" - and it absorbs from outside within and excretes from the body.

Not to mention, your skin is vital to the generation of vitamin D - which, as you grow older, becomes more difficult to generate as your skin loses this ability.

While it is true that you can use vitamin supplements, it has also been clinically proven that synthetically created vitamin D lacks some of the characteristics of naturally created vitamin D. Remember that going all natural whenever possible is the best course of action when it comes to keeping your body healthy.

Feet

Are you paying attention to your feet, and the shoes you are wearing? Many people, especially women, end up buying shoes for their looks, and pay a savage price for doing so later on. You should instead opt for comfort over vanity... your feet will thank you later.

Eyes

Are you taking proper care of your eyes? Be sure to have an additional source of light when you use your computer or television set. Additionally, stay away from cheap plastic sunglasses - they fail to remove the ultraviolet rays from the sun, whilst causing your eyes to be more sensitive because of the light being blocked out.

The damage caused is gradual but permanent. When you venture outside, protect your eyes with quality sunglasses - you only have one set of eyes!

Stomach

Your stomach is often just subjected to whatever you choose to consume, or whatever you feel like eating. The consumption of excessive caffeine - as found in coffee and some sodas - can systematically destroy the lining of your stomach, leaving you with ulcers or irritable bowel syndrome when you grow older.

These are just a few of the little things you should be attentive to, there are of course a number of other little things equally important- like your ears and how much noise you subject them to, your nails and whether they are allowed to breathe or just rot away underneath artificial nails, etc.

The little things that go unnoticed, that you don't pay attention to can often add up to poor health if not properly attended to. As a result your quality of life can be drastically reduced, just when you've become free to enjoy it.

There's a reason old age is called the "Golden Years", you are meant to live long and happily!

Are You Paying Attention to Your Weight?

You know, for most people, being reminded about taking care of their weight is quite irritating. They live busy lives, and do not always have the time to attend to their physical mass.

However, by not taking care of your weight, you could end up opening a whole can of worms one day - at a time in your life when you least want to have to deal with it!

When you are young *(below forty)*, the most serious thought that comes up when you think about your weight is the fact that you cannot wear your favorite clothes any more, or that your boyfriend or girlfriend will find you unattractive if you put on too much weight.

Some of us simply "accept our shortcomings" and live with it.

Unfortunately, being overweight is simply the beginning. The additional weight is merely an indication that something is wrong. It could be a slow metabolism, or maybe a poor eating pattern, or a problematic thyroid.

Whatever the cause of the excess weight, the real problem is the side effects that result from it.

The side effects of being overweight are numerous - ranging from problematic blood circulation and swollen limbs, to cholesterol, cardiac problems, and the increased likelihood of a stroke. Unfortunately, these side effects usually do not show up immediately, but their effects compound over time.

You will have to make a plan to deal with it whatever the cause of your unwanted weight. The risk involved is simply not worth it, and the drag of not being able to do what you want to do - physically - can be keeping you from enjoying many things in life right now.

Never mind what it will be like a few decades from now!

For most people, getting control of your weight is relatively simple:

a. Look at your eating habits. Consider what you eat, how much you eat, and when you eat it. Plan a decent balanced diet including vitamins and minerals, fiber, protein and energy. Stay away from excessive use of sugar, oily or fatty foods, unsaturated fat, and processed foods. Eat as much as you need - _not_ as much as you like.

b. Become more active by engaging in some mild form of exercise. There is - in most cases - no need to indulge in frantic strenuous exercise, since in most cases a regular brisk walk will do. In fact, if you are quite morbidly overweight it might be downright dangerous to exert yourself too much, since your body may not be able to meet what you suddenly demand of it.

c. Take a good look at your lifestyle, and consider your working hours, your sleeping hours, your stress levels, and how much - or little - relaxation you have in your life. A disorganized lifestyle without any sensible routine can make it difficult for your system to balance itself.

And we wouldn't want that now would we?

e You Getting Exercise, or Just Rushing Around?

u know this is somewhat sad, but there are so many people of the inion that their hectic lifestyles provide enough exercise for optimal alth. Unfortunately however, nothing could be further from the truth. In ct, it might very well be adding to the problem!

hectic lifestyle simply adds to stress. Stress, in turn, causes a "fight or ght" mode of operation - which means that a number of things in your dy change to facilitate it.

such, it actually *wears your body down* - without any benefits being rived from the process. Additionally, by not working on reducing stress, u will encourage conditions in which your body tries to store additional ergy in case it might need it in the near future and thus cause yourself gain weight instead of losing it.

the other hand, getting some *real* exercise holds some real benefits. one thing it will help you to maintain an increased metabolic rate, ich in turn will help you to keep your weight down. Additionally, the ysical exertion will help you to reduce stress, and work away your wanted frustrations.

other little known fact is that exercise can help you to sleep more undly. When you need to go to sleep, the internal temperature of your dy drops slightly, and returns to normal again when you wake up.

hen you engage in regular exercise, you actually *force* your body to crease its internal temperature while exercising - with the result that ere is a larger, more noticeable difference in temperature when your ological clock tells your body to switch off for the night.
e bigger the difference between your daytime and sleeping time ernal temperatures, the easier it will be for your body to shut down and t peacefully.

Exercise does not need to be strenuous to be beneficial. All that you need to do is to increase your heart rate a bit, increase your oxygen flow a bit, and work off some energy on the process *(which will, in truth, help to increase your metabolic rate)*.

Physical exercise could be any activity that you enjoy. It could involve going to the gym, or just a brisk walk around the park. It could involve swimming, cycling, aerobic exercises or any sport you enjoy. How you get the exercise is not important - but instead the fact that you *do get regular exercise*.

How much exercise you need will depend on many factors, including your age, the physical condition of your body, your weight, your lifestyle, stress levels, etc.

So if you lead a hectic lifestyle, you might just need more exercise than the person who does not simply because you need to get rid of the additional stress as well. Ultimately though any exercise is better than no exercise, so... get moving already!

Are You Getting Enough Sleep?

Common knowledge has led us to accept that the average person needs around eight hours of sleep per night. For some people it is just not convenient, and for others it is just not attainable - but what does it matter? How does it impact our health?

You might be forgiven for thinking that sleeping is merely a time of physical rest for the day ahead tomorrow. While that is part of the process, there is much more to it than that. Did you ever stop to think why you need to sleep?

By nature, your body can only handle so much physical endurance in one single day. While it is physically possible to push the limits from time to time, it cannot be done indefinitely without harmful side effects.

As you exert yourself during daytime, some processes in your body start lagging behind - pretty much like batteries wearing down - because energy is diverted elsewhere in the body as needed in the moment. When you sleep, these processes catch up on their backlog.

Additionally, your sleeping time is a time of healing. While sleeping, you do not apply any more pressure to parts of your body that may be unwell - like a broken rib, a head aching from stress, sore eyes, etc. With the pressure removed, the body can try to heal itself without interference or further damage.

And finally, sleeping time is when your mind is sorting itself out. During the first sleeping cycle (most people sleep in cycles of roughly three hours each), most of it is spent in a deep sleep to obtain as much physical rest as possible.

In the subsequent cycles, however, more and more of the sleeping time is devoted to what scientists refer to as "rapid eye movement" periods. It is believed that we dream during these periods; which explains why you usually wake from a dream in the morning, and seldom do so during the middle of the night.

Keep in mind that the amount of sleep you get is not the only thing to pay attention to - it is also about the quality of sleep involved. It is of no use sleeping for eight hours per night if you are uncomfortable, or go to bed on a full stomach, or if you are surrounded by noise.

Additionally, light makes it difficult for most people to switch their minds off when trying to sleep. Light stimulates the production of chemicals in your brain that literally "wakes it up" - so the less light you have intruding into your bedroom, the better the quality of sleep you will enjoy.

Also remember that regular exercise will help your body to maintain temperature cycles *(it does not stay perfectly constant as most people believe)*, and by forcing it higher during daytime, your body will be able to "shut off" better when you have to go to sleep. Is all this starting to sink in now and sound familiar?

Eat healthy, sleep healthy, exercise healthy... all ingredients of the recipe for longevity and living well!

Are You Doing Your Part to Slow Nature Down?

Well, this brings us to our final strategy in increasing health, longevity and living our best life possible. Hopefully you've gained some much needed perspective by now and are on your way to living many more years to come!

Aging is a natural process - just like your body chemistry. While some things are simply inevitable, there are still ways and means of slowing down the hands of time in some respects. When you uncover and apply these methods, it can help you to enjoy a better quality of life for a much longer time.

That said, probably the biggest single cause of bodily deterioration is oxidation. Oxygen molecules enter your body, but the way in which they were formed leave them in such a state that they try to bond with anything in their way, and oxidize it.

These molecules are referred to as "free radicals", and are responsible for the gradual deterioration of your physical body.

Ironically, you will note that you can often see people living at sea level - where oxygen is abundant - who seem "old" at a relatively young age. On the other hand, there are a few communities in the world where people (besides having escaped progress as we know it) grow very old and remain healthy at high ages - and all of these are situated high up in mountain ranges, where there is less oxygen going around.

Since we cannot reduce the amount of oxygen we need to live off, we need to reduce the effect it has on our bodies.

This can be done by taking antioxidants. While there are many potent antioxidants in the vegetables we consume, there are two that stand out above all others:

The second strongest antioxidant on the planet is the acai berry from the Amazon. You can find this in supplement form at your local health food store or even purchase acai juice to drink.

Ironically enough though, cacao in its pure natural form is even *better* than the acai berry; it beats it hands down when it comes to providing antioxidants that fight free radicals.

In its natural form, cacao contains a substance that gives it a slightly bitter taste which is removed when it is commercially processed. This exact substance contains the precious antioxidants in huge amounts.

So, when in doubt, consume plenty of antioxidants by consuming plenty of pure natural cacao; followed by a chaser of acai juice!

nal thoughts:

chieving longevity is ultimately a matter of mindset. If you are focused
 the short term and the pleasures you hope to obtain momentarily, or
e problems you want to solve immediately, you might lack the
rsistence to pursue the healthy lifestyle you need in order to live longer.

 the other hand, if you want to enjoy your present quality of life for as
1g as is physically possible, then you have to start taking steps to ensure
at your body is being cared as well as it possibly can be.

ngevity is not just a goal - it is a lifestyle. It's a lifestyle that will allow you
 preserve your body, your abilities and the quality of your life for as long
 the good Lord sees fit, keeping disease, undesirable medical conditions
d other problems at bay in the process.

d quite frankly, if you fail to see the benefits of preserving what you
ve now, you will inevitably pay the price someday, one way or another.
e only question left then to ask is when?

ote eat right, exercise, decrease stress, and remember to take care of
e little things, and you just might live long enough to appreciate the life
u were gifted with.

at pretty much wraps up this book on health and longevity hopefully
u've learned a lot and will take your new knowledge and apply it.
 your health!

y Walkins